ISBN: 1-4782-4961-7
ISBN-13: 9781478249610

Matthew 6:33

"Seek the Kingdom of God, above all else, and live righteously, and he will Give You everything You need."

ATTITUDE

The longer I live, the more I realize the importance of ATTITUDE on life!

Attitude is more important than Facts. Attitude is more than the past, than money, than circumstances, than failures, than success, than what people think, say, or do. It is more than appearance, giftedness, or skill. Attitudes will make or break the individuals that make up families, communities, and nations. The thing that is so remarkable about YOUR attitude is, WE HAVE A CHOICE EVERYDAY to decide the attitude we will embrace. That is POWERFUL. We should not take that power for granted. We cannot change the fact that people will act according to their understanding; however, there is something the individual CAN and MUST take charge of and that is our ATTITUDE! I am convinced that what happens to me is not as important as how I allow it to affect me.

I WILL TAKE CHARGE AND MASTER MY ATTITUDE EACH DAY!

HOW TO STAY YOUNG AND LIVE WITHOUT STRESS

1. Throw out nonessential numbers. This includes age, weight, and height. Let the doctor worry about them. That's why you pay him or her.

2. Keep only cheerful friends. The grouches pull you down.

3. Learning is forever. Keep learning. Learn more about the computer, crafts, gardening, whatever. Keep your brain on "go". An idle mind is the devil's workshop and the devil's name is Alzheimer's.

4. Enjoy the simple things of life. Smell that flower. Watch the sunset. Go to the ocean. These are your gifts. Enjoy.

5. Laugh often, long and loud. Laugh until you gasp for breath.

6. The tears happen. Life is not easy. Endure, grieve, and move on. The only person who is with us our entire life is GOD. Be ALIVE while you are alive. Live in the now.

7. Surround yourself with what you LOVE. Family, pets, keepsakes, music, plants, hobbies, whatever. Your home is your refuge.

8. CHERISH your HEALTH! If it is good, preserve it. If it is unstable, improve it. If it is beyond what you can improve, get help. Your Health is your true wealth!

9. Don't take guilt trips. Take a trip to the mall, to the next county, to a foreign country, but not to where the guilt is.

10. Tell the people you LOVE that you LOVE them, at every opportunity.

AND ALWAYS REMEMBER:

LIFE is not measured by the number of breaths we take, but by the MOMENTS that take our breaths away!

Like aging some things will happen naturally, but with new information and new technologies we can slow down or prevent the deterioration of our bodies. Hair loss can be prevented and restored.

RESTORE MY BEAUTIFUL HAIR!

THE ULTIMATE HOW TO GUIDE FOR WOMEN OF COLOR FOR PREVENTING HAIR LOSS AND HAIR THINNING!

"Why is my hair falling out"? A cry heard daily from women. One of the most traumatic issues for a woman to deal with in life is hair loss and hair thinning. There are more than 60 million women suffering from some form of hair loss. Now, here in your hands, RESTORE MY BEAUTIFUL HAIR women will have some proven solutions for prevention, restoration, and camouflaging hair loss.

HAIR LOSS PREVENTION

TABLE OF CONTENTS:

FOREWORD

This book is about you! Are you one of millions suffering hair loss or hair thinning? Now you have in your hands practical and proven solutions that could change the way you feel about yourself and your hair.Restore My Beautiful Hair is your how to guide to understand hair loss and what steps to take to do something about hair loss issues you may be suffering. You now have the tool you need to: http://RestoreMyBeautifulHair.com

The best start to preventing hair loss is to understand the basics of hair: what it is, how it grows, what system malfunctions can cause it to stop growing. And this book will cover the bases for you. Note that the contents here are not presented from a medical practitioner, and that any and all dietary and medical planning should be made under the guidance of your own medical and health practitioners. This content only presents overviews of hair loss prevention research for educational purposes and does not replace medical advice from a professional physician.

INTRODUCTION

Women consider their hair to be their crown of glory. A woman's hair is an extension of herself. You see the same self-image in little girls. Hair is powerful. Hair is strength. A woman hair represents the love she has for herself. For these reasons and more women will do anything to grow, maintain, and hold on to her beautiful head of hair. For this reason, I write this book. I hope to share some information that will help any women, young lady, or little girl suffering hair loss or hair thinning RESTORE their beautiful hair.

I looked at my master cosmetology license and realized I have been in this industry over 30 years. With my cosmetology license I have worked with every texture of hair there is. The one thing that I realized is everyone wants beautiful HAIR! I remember living in Lakewood, California in the early 90's and witnessing what I thought was the number one reason most women of color suffer hair loss and thinning, fibres in a bag sold as hair .I remember going into a warehouse where Hispanics were processing this fibres to sell as hair. Koreans had imported these fibres from China and the Koreans owned the manufacturing and process and warehouse. Once this fibres was processed it was then sold to Women of color. One day I knew I would share this experience because I knew things were changing for the hair industry. This warehouse was filled to the ceiling with brown shipping containers holding fibres most people call hair. This warehouse was half football field, containers stacked in ten per row to the ceiling. In Compton, California. What a sight in 1992. Do you want to restore your hair? Do you want to prevent hair loss? Do you want to prevent hair thinning? This book will help you ***Restore Your*** *BEAUTIFUL HAIR!*

What are Synthetic Fibres?

Synthetic Fibers are made from synthesized polymers or small molecules. The compounds that are used to make these fibers come from raw materials such as petroleum based chemicals or petrochemicals. These materials are polymerized into a long, linear chemical that bond two adjacent carbon atoms. Differing chemical compounds will be used to produce different types of fibers. Although there are several different synthetic fibers, they generally have the same common properties. Generally, they are known for being:

- Heat-sensitive
- Resistant to most chemicals
- Resistant to insects, fungi and rot
- Low moisture absorbency
- Electrostatic
- Flame resistant
- Density or specific gravity
- Pilling

There are several methods of manufacturing synthetic fibers but the most common is the Melt-Spinning Process. It involves heating the fiber until it begins to melt, then you must draw out the melt with tweezers as quickly as possible. The next step would be to draw the molecules by aligning them in a parallel arrangement. This brings the fibers closer together and allows them to crystallize and orient. Lastly, is Heat-Setting. This utilizes heat to permeate the shape and dimensions of the fabrics made from heat-sensitive fibers.

Synthetic fibers account for about half of all fiber usage, with applications in every field of fiber and textile technology. Although many classes of fiber based on synthetic polymers have been evaluated as potentially valuable commercial products, four of them - nylon, polyester, acrylic and polyolefin - dominate the market. These four account for approximately 98 per cent by volume of synthetic fiber production, with polyester alone accounting for around 60 per cent.

Now you know!

Hair is the fastest growing tissue of the body, made up of proteins called keratins. Every strand of hair is made up of three layers: the inner layer or medulla (only present in thick hairs); the middle layer or cortex, which determines the strength, texture, and color of hair; and the cuticle, which protects the cortex. Hair grows from roots, which are enclosed in follicles. Below this is a layer of skin called the dermal papilla, which is fed by the bloodstream carrying nourishments vital to the growth of hair. Only the roots of hair are actually alive, while the visible part of hair is dead tissue, and therefore unable to heal itself. It is vital then to take care of the scalp and body in order to perpetuate hair growth and maintenance. There are treatments and products formulated to help you maintain a healthy scalp and hair that will promote hair growth. These products and treatments will prevent hair loss and hair thinning. There has been major research done in this area because so many people have the problem. There is hope!

The most common type of hair loss seen in women is androgenetic alopecia, also known as female pattern alopecia or baldness. This is seen as hair thinning predominantly over the top and sides of the head. For women of color there is the issue of traction alopecia. This is seen as hair loss primary along the hairline, especially around the temples and above the ears. It is the result of tension caused by certain taunt hairstyles, weaves, braids, locs, ponytails, micro-braids and extensions.

These problems affect kids also and have more of a traumatic effect on their hair that has not fully developed. This problem is reversible when it first appears but left untreated, overtime the condition becomes permanent. Central Centrifugal Cicatricial Alopecia or hot-comb alopecia caused by excessive heat from hot combs, curling irons, and flat irons. Women with this condition experience hair loss or hair thinning mostly in the crown of the head. Hair becomes brittle and weak. CCA can cause scarring of the scalp. Some of the first warning signs are tenderness and inflammation. Left untreated, later signs include a shiny scalp and noticeable hair thinning. Chemical processing is another culprit that causes hair thinning and hair loss. Having the right information will prevent these problems for women and children of color.

Hormones called androgens, usually testosterone, can cause hair follicles to shrink, causing thinning of hair or eventual hair loss. Reportedly only bone marrow grows faster in our body than hair does. The average scalp contains 100,000-150,000 hair follicles and hairs, with 90% growing and 10% resting at any given time. Hair actually grows in three stages: anagen, catagen, and telogen. The anagen phase is the phase where hair is actively growing, and of course this phase is longer for follicles in the scalp than anywhere else on your body, and lasts longer for women than men. It is natural for follicles to atrophy and hair to fall out, and this is called the catagen phase. This phase is only temporary, and eventually the follicle enters the telogen phase where it is resting. These are the 10% at rest mentioned above. Normal anagen phases last approximately five years, with catagen phases lasting about three weeks, and telogen phases lasting approximately 12 weeks. As you see it is natural to lose some hair. Natural hair loss is considered to be in the range of 100 hairs per day. It is not apparent to most people that hair is actually being lost until more than 50% of a person's hair is actually lost.

More Hair Facts and Hair Loss Basics

Although both men and women can suffer significant hair loss, over 50% of men will suffer with Male Pattern Baldness (MPB), also known as androgenetic alopecia, at some point in their lives. The reason behind hair loss is a genetically inherited sensitivity to Dihydrotestosterone (DHT) and 5-alpha-reductase. The enzyme 5-alpha-reductase converts testosterone, a male hormone, to DHT, the substance identified as the end-cause for hair loss.

Most hair loss follows a pattern that has been codified in a table called the Norwood Scale (see figure 1). There are seven patterns of hair identified in the Norwood Scale, Norwood I being a normal head of hair with no visible hair loss, Norwood II showing the hair receding in a wedge-shaped pattern. Norwood III shows the same receding pattern as Norwood II, except the hairline has receded deeper into the frontal area and the temporal area. Type IV on the Norwood Scale indicates a hairline that has receded more dramatically in the frontal region and temporal area. Additionally there is a Additionally there is a balding area at the very top center of the head, but there is a bridge of hair remaining between that region and the front. Type V on the Norwood Scale shows that very same bridge between the frontal region and the top center, also called the vertex, beginning to thin. Type VI on the Norwood Scale indicates that the bridge between the frontal region and the vertex has disappeared. Finally, Type VII on the Norwood Scale shows hair receding all the way back to the base of the head and the sides just above the ears. Norwood patterns are determined genetically.

Norwood Scale Hair Loss for Men

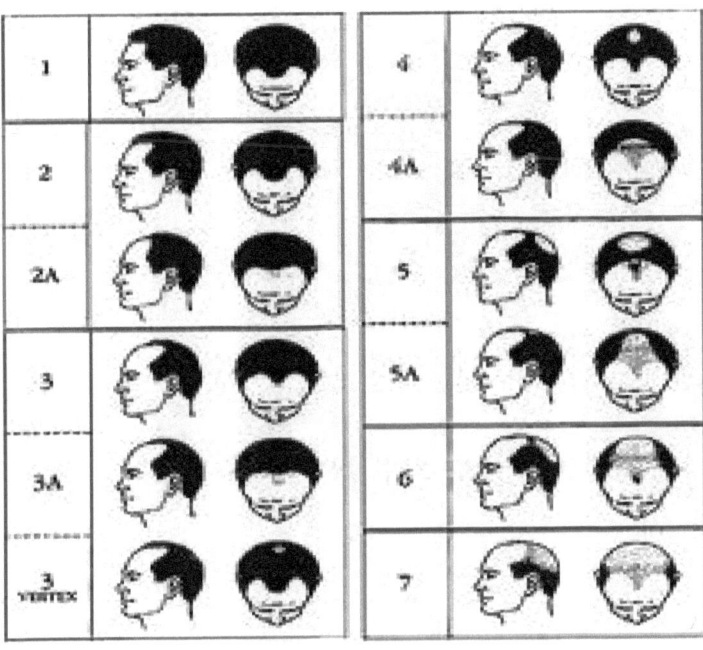

Traction Alopecia for women

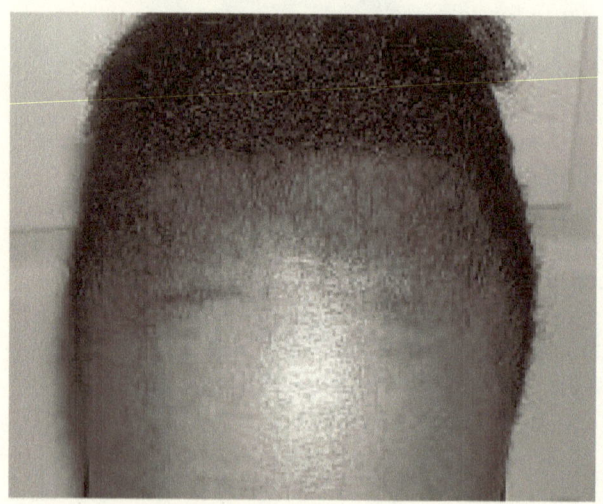

Traction Alopecia for little girls

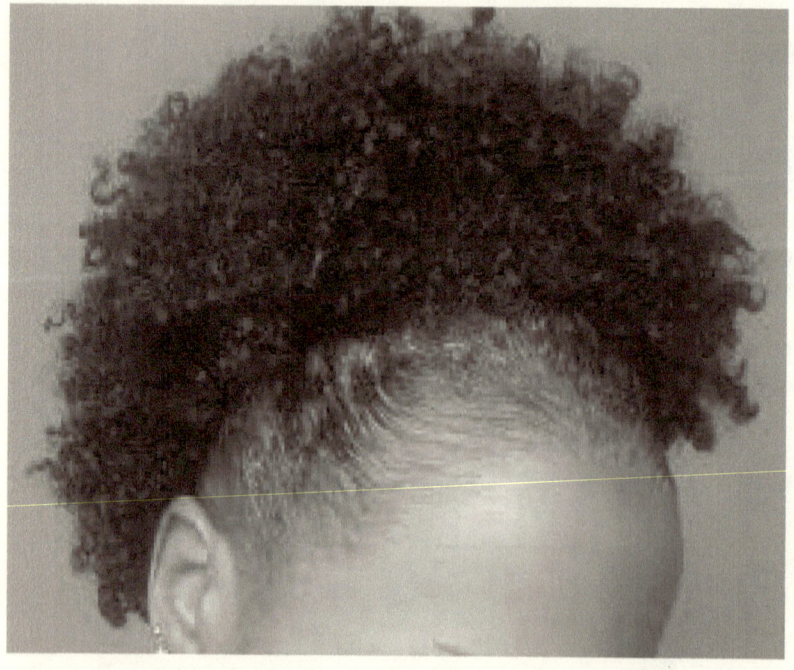

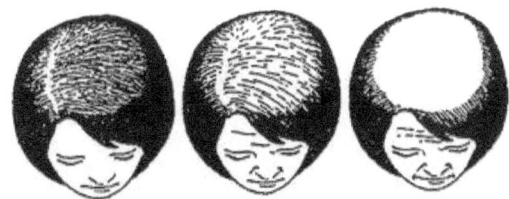

Female Pattern thinning and hair loss

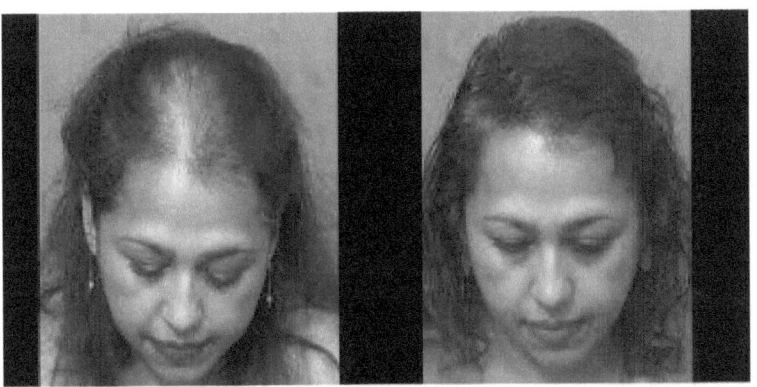

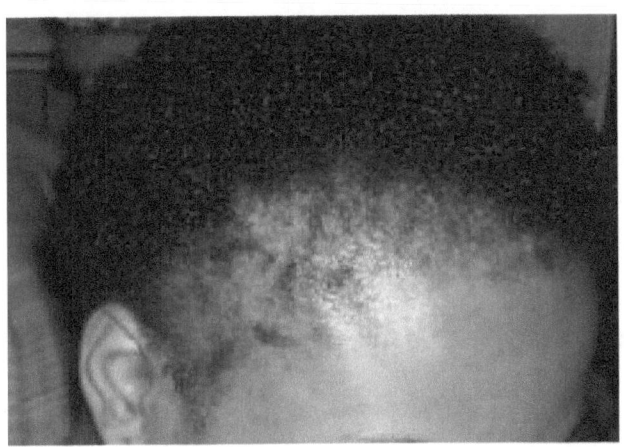

Hair loss has been noticed and studied throughout the ages, and some interesting discoveries were made in ancient times. For one it was noticed that eunuchs: those males without genitals-never went bald. Men who were castrated as a result of accidents in battle also never went bald. This was the first indication that testosterone had something to do with hair loss. It has also been found that the more recessive the hair gene, the more propensity toward baldness one has. Blond-haired persons have a greater propensity toward hair loss than darker-haired people, and therefore Caucasian persons have a greater propensity toward hair loss than non-Caucasian people. Beyond the genetic propensity of certain people toward hair loss, there seems to be various dietary triggers that activate the process, a notion that is promising since this can be controlled.

What exactly are androgens? Androgens are sex hormones mainly produced by males, the main one of which is testosterone. Androgens are produced by the adrenal glands, which protect the body in stressful situations by also producing adrenaline so that the body may respond to situations it deems to be threatening. The stress of daily life in Western civilization has caused a state of alarm in people that has made the body unable to distinguish between everyday stressors and threatening situations. Therefore the adrenal glands in most people in Western civilizations are overactive, constantly producing adrenaline and naturally producing testosterone along with it. Additionally, the over-consumption of red meat and high fat foods in Western society cause an overactive adrenal gland, perpetuating this situation.

There is a definite connection between the syndrome of Male Pattern Baldness (MPB) and the prostate gland. The prostate gland is actually a cluster of small glands in males surrounding the urethra, located just below the bladder. There is not a lot known discoveries were made in ancient times. For one it was noticed that eunuchs: those males without genitals-never went bald. Men who were castrated as a result of accidents in battle also never went bald. This was the first indication that testosterone had something to do with hair loss. It has also been found that the more recessive the hair gene, the more propensity toward baldness one has. Blond-haired persons have a greater propensity toward hair loss than darker-haired people, and therefore Caucasian persons have a greater propensity toward hair loss than non-Caucasian people. Beyond the genetic propensity of certain people toward hair loss, there seems to be various dietary triggers that activate the process, a notion that is promising since this can be controlled.

There is not a lot known about all the functions of the prostate, except that it serves to squeeze seminal fluid into and through the urethra during ejaculation. Prostate problems can cause serious problems with urination it becomes enlarged, and sometimes the prostate becomes cancerous. The syndrome of non-cancerous enlargement of the prostate is known as benign prostatic hyperplasia (BPH). DHT is responsible for the division of cells in the prostate, and is normally expelled by the prostate. However, when the prostate fails to expel the DHT, it builds up and causes enlargement. It has been confirmed that typical North American and northern European diets lend to the perpetuation of BPH and prostate cancer, whereas these are uncommon phenomena in other lands and was even uncommon here in the past. This is significant because the overproduction of DHT is responsible for BPH and prostate cancer, and is also responsible for MPB or androgenetic alopecia. The findings in research for BPH cures have usually simultaneously produced benefits in hair growth. We shall cover some of these discoveries in various sections of this book. Additionally, changes in diet are necessary to avoid all of these conditions and improve overall health.

Some common myths have arisen concerning hair loss. Because of medical advancements many of these myths are being addressed and corrected. For starters, although androgenetic alopecia or pattern baldness is genetic and therefore can be hereditary, it is not passed down through only your mother's side of the family. Either side of the family can pass down the genetic disposition toward baldness. Also, contrary to old family tales, wearing hats does not cause baldness either.

Most common hair loss comes under what has been commonly known as Male Pattern Baldness (MPB). Although referred to as MPB, females suffer a similar syndrome, so it is more properly called androgenetic alopecia. Although hair loss is not life or health threatening, it can cause serious problems with a person's psyche and self-confidence. There has been no absolute cure found for hair loss, and many factors of hair loss are hereditary, however there are several preventative measures one can take to maintain healthy hair and scalp.

A condition most people have never heard about is Trichotillomania. Trichotillomania is a disorder characterized by the non-cosmetic pulling of hair, resulting in significant hair loss. The name is derived from the Greek terms for hair (trich), pulling (tillo) and morbid impulse (mania). Trichotillomania (trich) occurs more frequently in women and is commonly associated with considerable distress. Hair is most commonly pulled from scalp, eyelashes, eyebrows, beard, and pubic area, though hair from any part of the body can be pulled. For more information check out the resources information at the end of the book.

DIET, NUTRITION AND HAIR LOSS

One key factor in maintaining a growing protein on a part of one's biological body is obvious: one must maintain a healthy diet. Although certain factors have been definitely identified as contributors to hair loss, we must keep in mind that hair is part of the complete biological system of the human body. Being a system, dysfunctions in one part of the system can contribute to dysfunctions in other parts; chain reactions occur when one part of the body malfunctions, causing other parts within the system to falter. To maintain optimum health, it is best to maintain a healthy diet and regular exercise regimen.

Defining exactly what a healthy diet is when it comes to preventing hair loss can be a little more complex. Principally, the main vitamins, minerals, and nutrients that one must ingest in some form to maintain healthy hair are vitamin A, all B vitamins-particularly vitamins B-6 and B-12, folic acid, biotin, vitamin C, vitamin E, copper, iron, zinc, iodine, protein of course, silica, essential fatty acids (EFA's, formerly known as vitamin F) and last but not least one must consume water. There are also certain foods that may cause dysfunctions that will contribute to hair loss.

The best way to maintain a healthy vitamin and mineral intake is a good diet. Supplements will help in maintaining a healthy scalp environment. It's not easy to maintain beautiful skin, hair, and nails in today's world. Everything from pollution to stress to UV rays adds to the challenge. ***NUTRILITE Complex for Hair, Skin & Nails*** will help you look your best. Fortunately, we also live in a time where scientific research is constantly discovering better ways to treat these problem areas. Discoveries like biotin – one of the main ingredients in ***NUTRILITE Complex For Hair, Skin & Nails***. This unique combination of nutrients provides a wider range of recognized support for these three problem areas than any other leading brand.

Benefits
Contains:
- Biotin, a B vitamin which may prevent nail brittleness and promote healthy hair and improve skin condition
- Collagen, a major structural protein of connective tissues
- Grapeseed Extract, a powerful antioxidant

- Glycine, an amino acid that works in conjunction with collagen to promote skin moisturization
- L-Cysteine, an amino acid that promotes the formation of keratin, a major protein in hair, skin and nails
- Horsetail Herb Extract, a natural source of silicic acid and silica, traditionally associated with healthy hair and nails
- Vitamin C, an important antioxidant

As a hairstylist I always recommended this product and clients had great results. I worked for one of the largest hair restoration companies in the world, yes the one you see on TV, and one of the services was hair and scalp treatments. Nutrition is the major part of restoring and maintaining your hair. Let's face, we can't get all nutrition from foods. The most important thing about this brand is that it is all natural. The joy is nutrition and maintaining a healthy scalp environment. Another product solution is ___Satinique Scalp Serum___. This product is used topically and is full of nutrition. Scientifically formulated to deliver fast-acting, leave-in protection that maintains your scalp's optimal health and helps safeguard hair structure. Completely nourishes scalp with vitamins (E, H, B, A), antioxidants, protein, and lipids. See an 83 percent increase in scalp hydration after just one hour and a 53 percent reduction in dry flakes in two weeks.

Benefits

- 84% increase in scalp hydration after just one hour.
- 53% reduction in dry flakes in just two weeks.
- After just one application leaves hair 70% easier to comb.
- Instant hair smoothness and hydration with every use.
- Allows scalp to maintain elevated hydration for up to 24 hours.
- Hair shows a significant increase in elasticity after just one application, giving it greater resistance to breakage and splitting.
- Gentle and safe for use on permed and colored or other chemically treated hair.
- Reduces dry, itchy feeling, leaving the scalp hydrated and nourished.
- Rinse-free formula – no wait time! Immediately proceed to styling.
- Allergy tested and dermatologically tested.
- 8, 6-ml individual-use bottles.

Beneficial Ingredients:

- **Calming Agent**
  Effective for soothing: Ginkgo biloba.

- **Protectants**
  These ingredients are valuable as they help the scalp help itself to maintain a natural protective barrier: Ceramide Infusion System, Trehalose, Vitamin A Retinyl palmitate, Vitamin C.

- **Antioxidants**
  Look at nature's wonders – vitamins and powerful plant extracts to fight environmental and free radical damage with antioxidant protection: Vitamin E Tocopheryl acetate, Vitamin C, Grape Seed extract, Toucha Tea extract, Olive Leaf extract.

- **Moisturizers**
  Luxurious moisturizers like these enrich and hydrate: Hyaluronic acid, Sodium PCA, Vitamin E Tocopheryl acetate, Vitamin B5 Panthenol, Essential amino acids.

- **Shine and Support**
  Help support and protect hair while leaving it hydrated, and boosting natural shine and luster: Vitamin H Biotin, Ceramide Infusion System/Active LA, Wheat protein, Vitamin B5 Panthenol, Vitamin E Tocopheryl acetate.

- B-vitamins work interdependently and therefore all levels of B vitamins need to be sufficient in order to maintain proper health. Vitamins B-6, folic acid, biotin, and vitamin B-12 are all key components in maintaining healthy hemoglobin levels in the blood, which is the iron-containing portion of red-blood cells. Hemoglobin's primary function is to carry oxygen from the lungs to the tissues of the body, so if these vitamins were deficient in one's body, then hair and skin would indeed suffer. Fortunately some of the tastiest foods contain these vitamins. Vitamin B-6 is found in protein rich foods, which is excellent because the body needs a sufficient amount of protein to maintain hair growth as well. Liver, chicken, fish, pork, kidney, and soybeans are good sources of B-6 and are relatively low in fat when they are not fried. Folic acid is found in whole grains, cereals, nuts, green leafy vegetables, orange juice, brewer's yeast, wheat germ, and liver again. Meat, fish, poultry, eggs, and other dairy products meanwhile provide healthy amounts of B-12. Biotin deficiencies are rare unless there is a severe case of malnutrition or a serious intestinal disorder, since a healthy gut produces biotin through good bacteria found there. Note: if you have a known intestinal disorder and are plagued by hair loss, ask your doctor about biotin deficiencies and possible solutions.

- Vitamin C is responsible for the development of healthy collagen, which is necessary to hold body tissues together. A vitamin C deficiency can cause split ends and hair breakage, yet this is easily reversible with an increase to normal vitamin C levels. Vitamin C can be found in foods such as fresh peppers, citrus fruits, melons berries, potatoes, tomatoes, and dark green leafy vegetables.

- Vitamin E is necessary to provide good blood circulation to the scalp by increasing the uptake of oxygen. Vitamin E is derived from foods such as green leafy vegetables, nuts, grains, vegetable oils, and most ready-to-eat cereals, which are fortified with vitamin E.

- Vitamin E deficiencies are rare in people in North America and Europe. In the rare cases of vitamin E deficiency, usually caused by the inability to absorb oils and fats, dietary supplements are available.

- Copper is a trace mineral that is also necessary in the production of hemoglobin. Hemoglobin as mentioned earlier is vital to the process of carrying oxygen to tissues such as the hair, and obviously hair is alive cannot grow without proper oxygen, yet it does not breathe as other components of our body do, because the oxygen must get to the shaft of the hair. Good sources of copper are liver again, seafood, nuts, and seeds.

- Another key mineral vital in the production of hemoglobin is iron. Iron is found in two forms, heme and non-heme; heme iron is much easier to absorb into the system. This is where the problem lies. Of course most people know that red meat is a good source of iron, however red meat is non-heme iron and is difficult for the body to absorb, as are many iron supplements. Good heme iron sources are green leafy vegetables, kidney beans, and bran. Additionally, one can increase the absorption of non-heme iron into the body by consuming non-heme food sources and vitamin C sources in the same meal.

- Zinc is another vital component to healthy hair, being that it is responsible for cell production, tissue growth and repair, and the maintenance of the oil-secreting glands of the scalp. It also plays a large role in protein synthesis and collagen formation. For this reason, zinc is important for both hair maintenance and dandruff prevention. Most Americans are deficient in zinc. Most foods of animal origin, particularly seafood, contain good amounts of zinc; oysters are particularly rich in zinc. Zinc is also found in eggs and milk, although in much smaller amounts. Zinc from sources such as nuts, legumes, and natural grains is of a different type than those found in animal sources and is not easily used by the body, although oats are a good source of zinc that is readily used by the body.

- Protein is found in most of the aforementioned animal source foods, particularly meats, fish, milk, cheese, eggs and yogurt. There is no need for a person eating the average Western diet to eat additional protein. Too much protein, even though hair is made of protein, will not improve hair growth and may cause other health problems.

- A challenge for vegans is to maintain healthy levels of protein, being that complete proteins containing all nine essential amino acids necessary are found mostly in animal sources. Legumes, seeds, nuts, grains and vegetables do not contain the same form of protein necessary for a healthy body. There is only one common non-meat source for complete protein, and that is the soybean. Fortunately, soybeans have been made into tofu and texturized vegetable protein (TVP) so that they can be made into various dishes. Additionally, one may eat from a wide variety of vegetable sources in order to obtain all the essential amino acids.

- Iodine is vital to the growth of hair. Sheep farmers long ago discovered that vegetation void of iodine due to iodine-depleted soil will adversely affect the growth of wool in sheep. Likewise, our hair needs iodine to grow. Iodine is synthetically added to table salt, however in this form it is not assimilated well into the body and can therefore cause iodine overload. An excess of iodine in the body can adversely affect the thyroid. It is best to use non-iodized salt and retrieve your iodine from natural food sources. These include seaweed, salmon, seafood, lima beans, molasses, eggs, potatoes with the skin on, watercress and garlic.

- One of the most difficult nutrients vital to hair growth to get in one's diet is the trace mineral silica. Silicon is a form of silicon and is the second most abundant element in the earth's crust, second only to oxygen. The Earth provides everything we need for health, and with silicon being so abundant, it would seem that there would never be a problem with silica deficiency. Unfortunately, trace minerals are rare in Western diets because our food is processed and our soil depleted by chemical treatments so often that trace minerals are lost. Silica is vital to the strength of hair, and although it will not necessarily stop hair from falling out from the follicle, it will stop hair breakage. It works by stimulating the cell metabolism and formation, which slows the aging process. Foods that are rich in silica are rice, oats, lettuce, parsnips, asparagus, onion, strawberry, cabbage, cucumber, leek, sunflower seeds, celery, rhubarb, cauliflower, and swiss chard. Note that many of these foods, particularly rice, are a large part of Asian diets and Asians tend to have the strongest and healthiest hair. Be sure to seek out all the above foods from sources that grow food organically, as this is vital to obtaining the trace minerals that are usually not present in North American soil and therefore not in American foods. Additionally these foods should be eaten uncooked, or in the case of rice-unwashed, as trace minerals are easily cooked and washed away.

- Essential Fatty Acids (EFA's) are fatty acids that are needed by the body yet not produced by the body. EFA's are a key component to healthy skin, hair and nails. Common skin diseases, such as those discussed later in this book like eczema and seborrhea, are in part caused by deficiencies in EFA's. Including deep-water fish such as salmon, sardines, mackerel, trout, or herring approximately three times a week will provide sufficient amounts of EFA's. However, if for some reason you cannot eat deep-water fish or have an extreme dislike for it, it may be necessary to take a supplement to obtain the required amount of EFA's.

- Last but not least, make sure to include the proper amount of water in your diet. Water is vital to proper hydration, which is necessary in order for all nutrients to be utilized properly by the body, not to mention the proper function of every cell in the body including hair follicles. The suggested amount of water intake daily is eight 8-ounce glasses of water a day, or 64 ounces a day.

- The effects of high-fat diets and the increase of DHT (Dihydrotestosterone), a chemical produced by the body found to cause hair loss, is not conclusive at this time. However, there does seem to be a connection; as societies that consumed relatively low-fat diets such as pre-World War II Japan experienced almost no pattern baldness, whereas in post-World War II Japan there is an increase in pattern baldness as their society consumes a higher fat diet. In fact, Asian and African men in their native countries traditionally suffer very little Male Pattern Baldness (MPB). Although when the same peoples come to North America, they begin to develop MPB. Because people of all races and ethnicities tend to develop MPB or androgenetic alopecia, yet do not exhibit these tendencies before moving to America, changes in diet may be a leading contributing factor. Diets high in fat do increase testosterone, which is the main component in DHT. More research needs to be done on this topic to reach conclusive evidence, although it certainly could not hurt to lower one's fat intake.

- Fiber is vital to making sure undigested food moves through the body and to the bowels properly. Failure of foods to move through the bowels in a reasonable amount of time can cause fermentation of undigested food in the bowels and blocking of nutrients being absorbed through the body. Beyond causing degrees of malnutrition, this can also cause a level of toxicity that will overwork systems in the body such as the adrenal glands and contribute to hair loss. Healthy amounts of fresh vegetables, fruits and legumes consumed daily will ensure a proper amount of dietary fiber.

- Although nutritional remedies were those that were discussed here, supplements can be used if one feels they are simply unable to eat properly due to work schedule or dislike of certain foods. Nutritional supplements containing these same vitamins and minerals can be taken, with the exception of water of course. Be sure to always take supplements that are naturally chelated, meaning that the supplements were developed in a natural base. This will ensure that the supplements you consume will be more readily absorbed in the body. There are some cautions to taking supplements of certain vitamins and minerals, particularly those that are fat-soluble because the body stores them.

Vitamin A, can be highly toxic and supplements of vitamin A should be avoided unless recommended by a doctor. It is best to achieve one's vitamin A requirements either by food or through a naturally chelated multivitamin. Also remember that smoking and second hand smoke can cause blocking of vitamin A assimilation, so it is best to avoid smoking and remove one's self from areas and situations where second hand smoke is present if at all possible Vitamin E supplements should always be taken at 400 i.u. per day to start and work your way up to 800 i.u. Always take vitamin E in its natural form, which is d'alpha tocopherol. Avoid taking vitamin E supplements in the synthetic form dl'alpha tocopherol, which is derived from petroleum and is less available for assimilation into the body. If you have high blood pressure or other serious illnesses, consult a physician before taking vitamin E supplements.

Zinc is one fat-soluble mineral that can cause harm if an overdose is taken. Zinc can rob the body of copper, mentioned above as a key nutrient in hair growth and health, not to mention in other functions of the body. Zinc supplements should be taken in low doses, such as 5mg at a time. These can commonly be found in the form of zinc lozenges designed for sore throats. There is a "trick" to tell if you are taking too much zinc. When the zinc levels in the body have surpassed the level that they can be used, a metallic taste begins to form. If you pay attention to the metallic taste, you will know when enough zinc has been consumed, and you can then stop consuming zinc immediately.

Iron supplements are not recommended unless a doctor has diagnosed you with a severe iron deficiency. If you do take an iron supplement, avoid ferrous sulfate, which you will find as the most common over-the-counter iron supplement in drug stores. Ferrous sulfate is hard for the body to assimilate, and because iron is not water-soluble it will sit in the body and can cause severe liver problems over time. Further, ferrous sulfate causes constipation, which can trigger a great deal more problems besides being extremely unpleasant. One iron supplement that does not contain ferrous sulfate is called Floradix and is available in both liquid and pill form.

Since there are so few foods to mention that are grown in North America and contain a good amount of silica, supplements may truly be needed. Horsetail is an herb that is a rich source of silica. It is highly important to never take horsetail directly however, or take a supplement made from unprocessed horsetail, as this herb can be toxic when ingested whole, ground, in tablets or capsules. Horsetail must be taken in an aqueous extract of the herb only. Ask someone at your health food store or someone knowledgeable about herbs to help you find this form. Silica gel is suspended in water, although it is not an aqueous solution and should be avoided. Nettle is also a good source of silica and Nettle Root Extract is readily available at health food stores.

Supplements of Essential Fatty Acids (EFA's) are easily found in most health food stores and even many supermarkets and pharmacies. These include Evening Primrose Oil, Wheat Germ Oil, Flaxseed Oil, Cod Liver Oil, and other oils from deep-water fish. It is not recommended to rely on Cod Liver Oil as a source for EFA's because it contains high levels of vitamins A and D, and the amount of Cod Liver Oil necessary to achieve proper amounts of EFA's would cause overdosing on these vitamins. The recommended supplements are Evening Primrose Oil and Flaxseed Oil. Both these oils are available in oil form or in capsules. Keep in mind that high amounts of saturated fat blocks the effectiveness of EFA's, counteracting their effectiveness, so there needs to be adjustments to your diet if there is a high amount of saturated fat in it.

Juicing is a natural way to obtain many of the vitamins, minerals, and trace minerals mentioned above. When using organic fruits and vegetables, juicing can provide quite a boost to the system and encourage the health of hair. Juices are very readily assimilable by the body and provide the same content as the whole food. Fresh juices have a high enzyme content, which is beneficial because these enzymes are stored by the body and can be used by the body when cooked foods that have been robbed of enzymes are consumed. Storing the juice or purchasing pasteurized juices from the store diminishes this benefit, although the benefits of the minerals and vitamins are usually still available. All the above-mentioned fruits and vegetables can be juiced to obtain the maximum benefit from them. A great deal of silica, sulfur, iron, and potassium for example is extracted from organic carrot juice. In fact, carrots being roots contain most trace minerals the body needs. The effects of carrot juice are enhanced when adding cucumber juice to it, because of its high silica and sulfur content. Organic spinach juice is highly recommended, as it is high in iron, vitamin A, and other vital vitamins and minerals; it is often combined with lettuce and carrot juice, two very good sources of silica and vitamin A. Non-organic spinach juice can be extremely high in pesticides and should therefore be avoided. Spinach juice should also be avoided if one suffers from kidney stones, as it contains a large amount of oxalic acid, which exacerbates kidney stone growth.

There are a number of foods and substances to avoid and limit the intake of. Substances such as alcohol, caffeine, sugar and nicotine can deplete the body of nutrients and raise adrenal levels, which will cause a chain reaction of producing more androgen and causing hair loss. High levels of saturated fat and cholesterol rich foods are also linked to increased DHT levels and their consumption should be limited. Additionally, common table salt has been linked to hair loss. And the average diet provides the recommended amount of sodium intake; therefore, salt should never be added to food. However, when using salt for seasoning during cooking, be sure to use salt with Iodine being that it is a nutrient that is vital to hair growth as well, unless you are a regular consumer of seafood, which contains high levels of Iodine.

Toxemia can cause a great deal of dysfunction in the body's systems, including hair-loss related illnesses such as eczema, psoriasis, seborrhea and possibly several others. It is vital for one to cleanse the body of impurities in order to maintain a healthy system and avoid such illnesses, as there are no cure for these illnesses beyond cleansing and the maintenance of a healthy diet to allow the body to heal itself. Regular cleansing should include a diet rich in fiber as mentioned earlier, and the use of added fiber such as provided by consuming psyllium husk as a bulking agent along with laxative agents. Although hair loss can be caused by many other variables, lack of proper nutrition will assuredly cause hair loss in many people. Fortunately, adopting a proper diet that includes the above nutrients can reverse hair loss caused by malnutrition. One thing for certain, regardless of whether your hair loss was caused by malnutrition or not, adopting a healthier diet will help the function of other areas of the body.

Solutions for hair thinning and hair loss

I can remember in the 80's we used an electrical hair stimulator to promote hair growth and it worked. Stimulating blood circulation helps heal and restore a healthy scalp and hair. The latest technology, **_Low Laser Light Treatments_** hair is now used to restore and promote hair growth. You can go to a hair loss clinic or do treatments in the convenience of your home. When used with products specifically formulated to restore and promote hair growth, low light laser treatments make hair restoration a no brainer. The Hair Loss Control Clinics, developed by doctors, use a multi-therapeutic approach with products good for scalp hygiene, good hair nutrition, blocking DHT (the most common cause of hair loss and thinning) to restore and prevent hair loss.

Prevention is important when talking about hair loss and hair thinning. If you can create a program or your stylist create this program where you can use services and products to maintain the health of your hair, scalp, and body maybe your chances of maintaining your hair will be greatly improved. I know because I have done it for clients in the past. There are more solutions.

Whether we're 12 or 55 with hair that is natural, relaxed, pressed and curled, locs, braided, short or long, doctors say we are losing our hair at alarming rates. Being apart of the industry, change has been so dramatic. If you have seen the *movie Chris Roc, produced, "Good Hair*," then you understand why our hair is Our Crown of Glory. We will do anything to keep that! Hair loss can be very traumatic both psychology and physically. The good news whether our challenges are man-made, woman-made, or genetic there are a host of new treatments and new technologies design to restore even the most frail and fragile strands. Here are some other treatments and technologies to help you win your *Hair Loss Battle.*

The term Male Pattern Baldness (MPB) tends to lay credence to the thought that hair loss is primarily a male problem. While males do lose hair more readily and tend to lose hair in sections, women suffer baldness and hair thinning also, except the thinning is more uniform throughout the head. With this is mind, women are better candidates for surgical hair replacement, weaving treatments, and hair units because large portions of the scalp are highly unlikely to be bald on a woman suffering with androgenetic alopecia. Traction Alopecia is characterized by loss of hair along the hair line, especially around the temples and above the ears. It is a result of tension caused by certain hair styles-weaves, braids, locs, and ponytails. This can be devastating for young girls because their hair has not developed thus are much weaker in those areas. This type of hair loss is irreversible and overtime leads to permanent hair loss. That is why sharing this information is powerful. **_We CAN_** prevent hair loss and hair thinning with the proper education. There are recommended for this type of hair loss and damage. Topical hair serums that contain nutrients and other ingredients, strengthen, moisturize and protect those areas that are weaken by this type of hair styles. **_Satinque Hair Serum by Amway_** is one such product I have used and recommend. **Because it is** scientifically formulated to deliver fast-acting, leave-in protection that maintains your scalp's optimal health and helps safeguard hair structure. Completely nourishes scalp with vitamins (E, H, B, A), antioxidants, protein, and lipids. See an 83 percent increase in scalp hydration after just one hour and a 53 percent reduction in dry flakes in two weeks.

Benefits
- 84% increase in scalp hydration after just one hour.
- 53% reduction in dry flakes in just two weeks.
- After just one application leaves hair 70% easier to comb.
- Instant hair smoothness and hydration with every use.
- Allows scalp to maintain elevated hydration for up to 24 hours.
- Hair shows a significant increase in elasticity after just one application, giving it greater resistance to breakage and splitting.
- Gentle and safe for use on permed and colored or other chemically treated hair.
- Reduces dry, itchy feeling, leaving the scalp hydrated and nourished.

- Rinse-free formula – no wait time! Immediately proceed to styling.
- Allergy tested and dermatologically tested.
- 8, 6-ml individual-use bottles.

Beneficial Ingredients:

- **Calming Agent**
  Effective for soothing: Ginkgo biloba.

- **Protectants**
  These ingredients are valuable as they help the scalp help itself to maintain a natural protective barrier: Ceramide Infusion System, Trehalose, Vitamin A Retinyl palmitate, Vitamin C.

- **Antioxidants**
  Look at nature's wonders – vitamins and powerful plant extracts to fight environmental and free radical damage with antioxidant protection: Vitamin E Tocopheryl acetate, Vitamin C, Grape Seed extract, Toucha Tea extract, Olive Leaf extract.

- **Moisturizers**
  Luxurious moisturizers like these enrich and hydrate: Hyaluronic acid, Sodium PCA, Vitamin E Tocopheryl acetate, Vitamin B5 Panthenol, Essential amino acids.

- **Shine and Support**
  Help support and protect hair while leaving it hydrated, and boosting natural shine and luster: Vitamin H Biotin, Ceramide Infusion System/Active LA, Wheat protein, Vitamin B5 Panthenol, Vitamin E Tocopheryl acetate.

Because of ingredients you create a healthy scalp and hair environment for restoring healthy hair and scalp. Using a great scalp cleanser is very import! Eliminates chlorine, excess oil, and up to 100 percent of styling product buildup. daily on oily hair or, for other hair types, alternate with any of our other Satinique® cleanser/shampoos. Up to 167 uses.

Benefits

- Removes buildup from styling products, excess oil, and chlorine.

- Contains the Ceramide Infusion System, which replaces lost ceramide by penetrating each hair shaft, re-bonding and sealing it. Actually mends split ends and protects hair from future damage.
- Safe for chemically treated hair.
- Minimizes fading of colour-treated hair due to shampooing.
- pH balanced.
- Allergy tested.
- Dermatologically tested.

Using a great scalp cleanser is very important and Satinique products work and a little goes a long way. Need more information http://amway.com/georgegreen.

Because a great deal more emphasis is put on the beauty of a woman's hair, this is becoming a great concern for today's woman. While the general information covered thus far is good for all persons in general, there are a few things specific to women concerning hair loss.

Many women suffer hair loss and an increase of facial hair after the onset of menopause. This is because of the drop in estrogen production, changing the ratio of estrogen to testosterone in a woman's body. Prior to menopause, a woman's body is constantly producing estrogen, which binds excess testosterone to proteins called globulins. Therefore, there is little excess testosterone in a woman's body. After the onset of menopause this estrogen is no longer present, thereby exposing it to a similar although milder type of syndrome that males go through concerning the overproduction of DHT. An interesting note is that once again, the syndrome of menopause and its unique effects are not as common in the Eastern world, but are specific to Western civilization. The key differences are the consumption of less red meat and fatty foods in Eastern lands than in the West and less daily stressors in most Eastern lands as compared to Western civilization.

Anorexia is an eating disorder that is becoming more prevalent among women in the past few decades and is psychologically driven in Western society due to the emphasis put on slender women being the ideal in Western civilization. Needless to say, if you or a loved one is suffering with this disorder, a qualified physician should treat any cases of anorexia. However, some of the side effects of anorexia can be hair loss due to the malnutrition the syndrome caused. In this case, it is vital to carefully follow the advice given in the sections Nutrition, Diet, and Hair Loss, and Natural Hair Remedies.

It is of course recommended in all cases that you reduce your intake of red meats, fatty foods, and reduce stress, however due to your profession and engrained habits there may be a limit to how much you can change this part of your lifestyle. There is another factor in Eastern civilizations that may cause a stark difference in their women not suffering through typical menopausal symptoms here in the West. The consumption of soybeans and soybean products is much higher in the East. This is significant because soy contains estrogen-like substances and work in the body similarly to estrogen. Therefore there is not an extreme drop in estrogen levels in women who consume soybean products, thus reducing the symptoms of menopause typically suffered in the West.

Some women who suffer hair loss tend to have gastrointestinal problems that do not allow them to absorb proteins and zinc that are necessary to maintain a healthy head of hair. If you think that you have problems with your gastrointestinal system and are experiencing unusual hair loss, of course see your doctor. You may be able to take some natural non-dairy acidophilus after meals for a couple of months in order to increase your digestion of these nutrients.

There are a number of myths associated with hair loss in women particularly. Many were told that brushing the hair 100 strokes each night will promote healthy hair growth. As mentioned earlier, extreme brushing of the hair can cause stress on the hair which can cause breakage and hair loss. Also, just as hats have been rumored to cause hair loss, wearing wigs has also been rumored to cause hair loss. This is very untrue, especially if the scalp is given sufficient time to breathe at night and hair is washed regularly to avoid buildup. Although stress can cause temporary hair loss, permanent hair loss is usually unconnected to stress. Last but not least, the belief that there are cosmetic products that are out on the market that grow hair is simply unfounded. There is only one product on the market that has been proven to grow hair on women safely, and that is women's Rogaine® discussed later in the section over the counter treatments.

During pregnancy hair growth increases dramatically in most women. This increases the usual percentage of hair normally growing on the head. Therefore, after childbirth there may be an increase in hair loss due to more hair follicles than usual entering the rest phase. The temporary excessive loss of hair usually occurs between one and three months after childbirth and is quite normal; it should balance out a few months after childbirth at most. Similar syndromes occur after ceasing birth control pills or switching types of birth control pills.

HAIR REPLACEMENT AND RESTORATION TECHNIQUE

Hair Today, Gone Tomorrow...HAIR RESTORATIONS SOLUTIONS for hair thinning and hair loss

Hair Today, Gone Tomorrow...HAIR RESTORATIONS SOLUTIONS for hair thinning and hair loss.

NEWS: Emory Facial Center hair restoration procedure featured on CBS Atlanta Discussion of hair restoration options for women experiencing thinning hair and hair loss.

If you're experiencing thinning hair or baldness, you're not alone. Hair loss is the single most common aesthetic complaint among men, affecting 40 to 50 million men in the United States. While it is less talked about among women, 20 to 30 million women in the United States also suffer from hair loss. The Emory Facial Center has the solution.

Dr. Ken Anderson specializes in the medical and surgical treatment of hair loss, providing platinum-level, one-on-one service to his patients. He is one of a select few surgeons in the U.S. trained in follicular unit extraction (FUE), an innovative technique that requires no incisions or sutures and leaves no scarring. During surgery, Dr. Anderson removes and relocates hair one follicle at a time. As a result, hair restoration looks and feels natural, without plugs or lines. And Dr. Anderson's techniques ensure your comfort throughout the procedure and reduced downtime afterwards.

Because everyone's hair-loss pattern is different, Dr. Anderson designs hair restoration plans that are unique to the individual. He'll not only address your current concerns; he'll work with you long term to ensure the ongoing health of your hair.

Dr. Anderson is certified by both the American Board of Otolaryngology (Head & Neck Surgery) and the America Board of Facial Plastic and Reconstructive Surgery. He also has formal training in the fine arts and combines his artistic talents with extensive experience to bring patients outstanding permanent results. To learn more about Dr. Anderson, contact Emory Facial Center and Hair Restoration, Atlanta, Georgia.

For more information make comment or call 678-818-4333.You should follow http://greenwayz.com for latest great information.

This procedure will help many, many, people. The secret is to get help early. Your hair care professional is your first line of defense. You concerned about what is happening to your hair, ask questions.

This information is great too if you are suffering hair loss or hair thinning. This is a great solution!

Coconut oil is traditional oil that people in tropical places have used for hundreds of years to condition and maintain healthy hair. Countries like India have entire industries based around coconut oil for hair treatment.

In recent years, coconut oil has been popularly used for natural hair treatment with African hair types. Audrey Sivasothy, a writer on the Yahoo associated content network, has done research on "Black Hair Care" and notes that coconut oil is an excellent choice for a pre-treatment before the hair is shampooed, as well as an excellent sealant on dry hair. She writes: "Many black women suffer from hair porosity issues as a result of our styling choices. Coconut oil's ability to prevent protein loss and reduce hair porosity makes it valuable oil for those who chemically relax, regularly straightens with heat, or permanently color their hair." Those in the "natural hair" movement have repeatedly testified to the benefits of switching from harsh chemical treatments to pure coconut oil. Their testimonials in public places like Twitter are very numerous. Sivasothy comments:

Coconut oil is a very unique hair oil. This versatile, low molecular weight oil is able to leverage its traditional oil status to seal the hair, but complements this sealing capacity with a strong affinity for hair proteins not found in other hair oils. Coconut oil benefits black hair in two important ways. First, coconut oil's hydrophobic oil characteristics allow it to inhibit the penetration of water from the surrounding air and environment. Second, coconut oil is able to bind to the natural protein structure of the hair. This helps the hair retain its natural moisture content and reinforces the hair fiber, making it stronger

Follicular unit extraction (FUE), also known as **follicular transfer** (FT), is one of two primary methods of obtaining follicular units, naturally occurring groups of one to four hairs, for hair transplantation. The other method is called strip harvesting. In FUE harvesting, individual follicular units are extracted directly from the hair restoration patient's donor area, ideally one at a time. This differs from strip-harvesting because, in strip harvesting, a strip of skin is removed from the patient and then dissected into many individual follicular units. The follicular units obtained by either method are the basic building blocks of follicular unit transplantation (FUT).

History and research

Follicular unit extraction (FUE) was first described by Masumi Inaba in Japan in 1988 who introduced the use of a 1-mm needle for extracting follicular units. Research into it was conducted throughout the 1990s. In 2002 it was first described in the medical literature by William R. Rassman and Robert M. Bernstein in their publication "Follicular Unit Extraction: Minimally Invasive Surgery for Hair Transplantation Robotic FUE devices were discussed at the 2007 meeting of the International Society of Hair Restoration Surgery (ISHRS), and research in robotic devices was presented by Dr. Miquen G. Canales and Dr. David Berman at the 2008 meeting of the ISHRS.Research was conducted by Restoration Robotics in Mountain View, California and the Berman Skin Institute in Palo Alto and found that follicles could be removed individually at a rate of up to 1000 per hour through the use of 1-mm hollow needles. Despite showing evidence of improvements in the transection rate versus the prior year's discussion, the findings suggested that transection at a rate of 6–15% was not low enough for general use in hair restoration procedures.

There are still extremely few surgeons and practices which have mastered Follicular unit extraction because the procedure takes considerable time and expense to learn and to develop skills to a high standard.

Follicular unit survival

The survival of follicular units upon extraction from the scalp is one of the key variables of successful hair transplantation. If follicular units are transected in the extraction process, there is a greater likelihood that they will not survive the transplant, and the hair transplant will fail. While FUT procures using strip-harvesting of follicular units typically guarantees a large number of non-transected follicular units, FUE procedures can, and often do, transect grafts, rendering them useless in a transplant. Significant efforts have been made to reduce the rate of transection in FUE procedures. The skill of the surgeon and his/her team, and the type of instrumentation used, are major factors in the ultimate yield and viability of the follicular units.

Scarring

FUE harvesting of grafts causes "pit" scarring; small, round, and typically white scars; in the patient's donor area where the grafts have been removed. FUE scarring differs from scarring from strip harvesting in that the latter procedure produces a linear scar in the donor area where the strip of skin was removed. Both the pit scarring from FUE and linear scar from strip harvesting are often hard to detect when hair in the donor area is at a normal length and the extraction is performed by a skilled surgeon. While the outcome of the healing process, and thus the appearance of scar tissue, depends on several variables; including the type of extraction, the skill of the surgeon, and, in strip harvesting, the method of wound closure; in both FUE and FUT, short cropped hair or a shaved head will typically reveal some scarring.

Comparisons with Follicular unit transplantation

Follicular unit extraction generally has a quicker patient recovery time and significantly lower post-operative discomfort than follicular unit transplantation (FUT). FUE provides an alternative to FUT when the scalp is too tight for a strip excision and enables a hair transplant surgeon to harvest finer hair from the nape of the neck to be used at the hairline or for eyebrows.

However, with FUE, the follicles are harvested from a much greater area of the donor zone compared to FUT, estimated to be eight times greater than that of traditional strip excision so requires patients to have hairs trimmed in a much larger donor area. As a result, the hair in the lower and upper parts of the donor area, where the grafts were taken from, may thin and this can make the donor scars visible. Follicles harvested from borderline areas of the donor region may not be truly "permanent," so that over time, the transplanted hair may be lost. Maximum follicular unit graft yield is lower than with FUT and may result in greater follicular transection (damage). Due to the scarring and distortion of the donor scalp from FUE it makes subsequent sessions more difficult, and grafts are more fragile and subject to trauma during placing, since they often lack the protective dermis and fat of microscopically dissected grafts, ultimately which may result in poor growth. A problem of buried grafts can occur during the blunt phase of the three-step technique when the graft is pushed into fat and must be removed through a small incision. FUE can also more expensive and take longer to perform than FUT, so grafts are usually out of the body longer, risking sub-optimal growth.

There has been a great deal of progress in the field of hair replacement and restoration in the past few years. Surgical techniques have improved greatly from the days when hair replacement first began. All hair replacement techniques involve the use of your own hair; therefore, hair replacement candidates must have some healthy hair, usually at the back and sides of the head. The process is a relatively safe procedure when performed by a qualified surgeon, however as with any surgery there are risks. Candidates must be checked for uncontrolled high blood pressure, blood-clotting problems, or skin that scars excessively, as these conditions may make healing difficult. There are solutions and this is one that is permanent and has great results.

Of course surgery is a serious option, and often an expensive one as well. For those not wishing to undergo surgery for either reason, the option of non-surgical hair additions is often explored. Many professionals have developed techniques to add hair to existing hair on your scalp that look very natural. Weaves, fusions, bonding, cabling and micro linking are some of the techniques used to bond hair to the existing hair or scalp non-surgically.

Many jokes were made in the past about wigs and toupees, and they have gained an unfavorable light amongst many people because they were so obvious on the wearer. Today's toupees and wigs are often made of real hair and are very well styled, causing them to look more natural on the wearer. These hairpieces are held in place by affixing adhesive to the scalp and stay in place through vigorous exercise. Of course you will need to seek a professionally made toupee in order to make it worth your while, and you should purchase at least two so that you can maintain them properly, servicing one while wearing the other. A professionally styled and fitted toupee is expected to cost upward of $600 to $1000 in today's market. Of course no one wants to go through the embarrassment of wearing the obvious "rug" on top of your head, so if you are not willing to spend the money it takes to purchase a professional toupee then it is probably best to not wear any hairpiece at all. Non-surgical hair services are very popular today. Companies like the Hair Club and Bosley offer solutions for women. Professional salons offer hair units for women hair loss suffers. Lace front units are very popular and look natural. You can purchase units made from human hair that will last 2-3 years with proper care. Extensions Plus a hair replacement store in Los Angles is known as the hair store for the stars. I remember a news report Cher the singer lost a $10,000 hair unit. I'm sure she had insurance. When it comes to looking good and feeling great, your hair has to be right. Cost, well whatever your hair has to be RIGHT!

A much safer procedure is hair weaving, yet this can only be used if hair is thinning and large balding areas are not present. The process is also called hair intensification or hair integration. When done properly weaves give your hair the opportunity to rest. Weaving can be a great way to grow your hair with the proper care. Care must be given to your scalp. Making sure your scalp is properly cleaned and moisturised. When wearing any type of extension it is very important to invest in hair that is 100% human hair. Tip~ real human hair will cost more than$25-$45. It is highly recommended that you consult with a hair care professional when investing in human hair. I can remember leaving the salon one day and noticed this lady with a hair style that was becoming on her. To my surprise I just commented to the other stylists her hair looked plastic! After thinking about what I had just said I told them that this lady hair style was plastic! When you go to most beauty supply stores what you are really buying is a plastic fiber. That is right PLASTIC. This fiber has been marketed as human hair, 100% human hair. ***NO LYE, THAT IS A LIE!*** Recently burglars have been breaking into beauty supply stores stealing what they think is real hair. That is what we have all been told. Truth is this is a plastic fiber that will cut your hair. This is another reason we have hair loss epidemic. Most people have never seen what I saw that day in a warehouse in Compton, California. Barrels and barrels of FIBER being process and sold to women of color, as 100% Human Hair. When you need help be sure you ask someone that knows how to properly do these services.

It is highly recommended that one seek professional assistance with these procedures from licensed hair professionals or barbers, and have a patch test done to the skin if using adhesives to test for skin sensitivities. Extra care must be taken to maintain cleanliness of the hair and scalp when wearing added hair in order to maintain the health of existing hair and the scalp in general. Of course, if you are undergoing chemotherapy or are in the early stages of diagnosed alopecia areata then these procedures should be avoided as the hair they are connected to is likely to fall out as well. Either waiting for a period of time or obtaining a full prosthesis is recommended in these cases.

Yet still there is another type of treatment which is a spray of micro fibers made up of the same substance that hair is made of: keratin. If your hair is simply thinning, while you are investigating a more permanent solution to your hair loss problems or in the process of employing a particular process that takes some time, you can use these substances to cosmetically produce the appearance of thicker and fuller hair. The substance is marketed under several different names, one such being Topik®. Being a temporary solution it is relatively inexpensive, and can provide some immediate aesthetic results to bolster confidence and optimism as you work on more permanent solutions.

OVER THE COUNTER TREATMENTS

The most popular over-the-counter hair restoration drug today is Rogaine®, a brand of topical monoxidil solution by Pfizer Corporation, approved for over the counter sale in 1997 by the Food and Drug Administration (FDA). Monoxidil was originally used as a blood pressure medication, and then doctors found that it produced the side effect of increased scalp hair growth. Today monoxidil remains the only FDA approved pharmaceutical topical solution proven to grow hair. In the preliminary studies held in 1985, 55% of men tested were able to re-grow hair with extra strength Rogaine® (5% topical monoxidil treatment), although the best results came from those who had been balding for less than 10 years and were bald in a section of four inches across or less. Another test study compared the results of regular strength Rogaine® (2% topical monoxidil solution) with the extra strength version, and found that subjects grew 45% more hair with the extra strength Rogaine® than with the regular strength Rogaine®, and users of both solutions outgrew the users of the placebo. Only 6% of those tested experienced any type of irritation. Rogaine® works by blocking the production of DHT. Of course there are generic brands of topical monoxidil solution also on the market. Rogaine® was originally made only for men's use, and then a women's version of the drug was produced. Similar results were achieved with the women's version. As with both men's and women's versions, users must take note that continuous use of the drug is necessary to maintain the newly grown hair, as it is a usual reaction for newly growing hair to stop growing and fall out when one ceases to use the drug. As with any drug, follow all directions and cease to use if irritation or discomfort persists.

Of course many people choose not to use drugs to treat conditions, because they want to avoid the use of chemicals and their possible side effects. In this case, there are several treatments in existence that have been found to block the production of DHT and thus work similarly to topical monoxidil products. As mentioned earlier, Saw Palmetto has been used effectively to block DHT in the treatment of prostatic disease, and is now being explored for its effectiveness in stimulating hair growth. Traditionally it has been used by herbalists to stimulate hair growth effectively. Nettles, usually taken in the form of Nettle Root Extract have shown itself to be effective in preventing hair loss as well. More information on these was covered in the section called Natural Hair Remedies.

PRESCRIPTION DRUG TREATMENTS

While topical solutions such as Rogaine® brand monoxidil have been used to treat hair loss, Propecia® brand Finasteride by Merck & Company, Inc. is the only FDA approved pill approved for the prevention of hair loss and possible hair re-growth. Like Rogaine®, Propecia® was discovered when its generic equivalent being used for another purpose was found to have beneficial side effects. Finasteride is the generic name for the drug, which was already in existence for quite some time and had been produced under the name Proscar® by Merck & Company and used for treatment of enlarged prostates, a syndrome medically called benign prostatic hyperplasia (BPH). BPH is caused by an overproduction of DHT, which causes the prostate to grow. Many BHP patients were also suffering with MPB, and when patients began taking Proscar®, they noticed the re-growth of hair also. This sparked new testing and the birth of Propecia® as a hair restoration drug. The approval of Propecia® by the FDA was easy to achieve, since it was merely marketing already approved Finasteride as a hair restoration drug, with a much smaller dosage than that required for BPH.

Propecia® is being prescribed by doctors to some patients as an oral treatment to internally block the production of DHT. Propecia is an androgen hormone inhibitor only approved for men, and has been clinically proven to grow hair on a significant percentage of men who suffer with Male Pattern Baldness (MPB) or more properly androgenetic alopecia. Unfortunately, the drug has not been approved for use by women at this time. This is especially true for women who are pregnant or can become pregnant, because the process of inhibiting testosterone from being converted to DHT can affect secondary sex characteristics of unborn fetuses.

Propecia® works by reversing the shrinkage of hair follicles that are in the telogen phase, or last phase of the normal hair cycle. Propecia® works best in combination with topical treatments of Monoxidil such as Rogaine®. Participants in studies have seen hair grow in as little as six months, whereas those who have seen no results in a year's time are reported not likely to see any results from the drug. One round of testing of over 2,000 men with androgenetic alopecia over a four-year period showed half with reported new hair growth.

Side effects of Propecia® in a few persons studied include diminished sex drive, difficulty in achieving an erection, and a decreased sperm production. Side effects were found in less than three percent of participants in clinical studies. Fortunately when the drug's use was discontinued, the side effects went away and normal functions resumed. Of course there are some who say that the growth of new hair is worth the cost of a drop in libido. Only you can decide whether this side effect is worth the personal cost to you. Finasteride is metabolized primarily by the liver, and therefore anyone suffering with liver disease may not be able to take the drug, and should consult a physician. Additionally, as with Monoxidil, it can mask PSA levels, thus caution should be used if used by patients with elevated PSA levels, as it may be difficult to read levels properly when diagnosing potential prostate cancer. Of course proper consultation with your physician will help determine if taking Finasteride treatments such as Propecia® is right for you.

An interesting phenomena concerning Propecia® is the dramatic rise in price it caused for Finasteride when it entered the market as a hair restoration drug. Propecia® is simply a 1mg version of Finasteride, a drug that was already being marketed as Proscar® for BPH by the same company that markets Propecia®, Merck & Company, Inc. Therefore there should not be an increase of any kind in the cost of production of Finasteride, since it was simply being marketed under a new name at a much smaller dosage. Merck & Company therefore was prepared to introduce Propecia at the price of $1.25 per pill or $37.50 for a 30-day supply in 1998. However, after reconsiderations it was decided that Propecia would be introduced at $50 for a one-month supply. This is compared to a 30-day supply of Proscar® which is 5mg Finasteride being marketed at $55-60.00 for a 30-day supply. The price was adjusted to be in the range of Rogaine® Extra Strength. The price of Propecia® today in 2004 is in the range of $130 for a 30-day supply, while Proscar® prices have risen at a much slower pace, and is now less expensive than the same Finasteride drug that is 1/5th the dosage. Doctors of course are discouraged by pharmaceutical companies to prescribe Proscar for cosmetic treatment of androgenetic alopecia. Of course there are always going to be those who find ways to circumvent this. Therefore, many have been driven to find ways to purchase Proscar®.

SUMMARY

Hair is a living protein, and as with any living part of our bodies we must be sure to maintain proper health to optimize our chances of maintaining a healthy head of hair. Proper nutrition is vital to maintaining healthy hair, since the hair is a living and growing part of the body's system. Viewing it in this manner can help us to treat our bodies different and raise expectations through proper care. A healthy balanced diet, occasionally with the help of vitamin and mineral supplements and exercise are all key components to a healthy regimen of maintaining healthy hair.

It is estimated that millions of women suffer some form of hair and hair thinning. Female pattern hair loss is the number one cause. Until solutions have been less than desirable. Now you are armed with practical information that will empower you against your fight against hair loss and hair thinning. Women want to live their lives to their fullest potential. With this information we have shared you can be sure you will be able to ***Restore Your Beautiful Hair*** and your confidence.

The scientific developments of the past two decades have brought hope and promise to many who suffer with hair loss. Treatments like Rogaine®, Rogaine® for Women, Propecia, and improved surgical treatments have brought relief to many who would have previously had to settle for gradual hair loss, wigs, or hairpieces. The discovery of the role of DHT in preventing hair loss has even opened the doors to possible herbal solutions to hair loss prevention, such as saw palmetto, nettles, rosemary and horsetail. Even more promising is the fact that the hair loss commonly known as androgenetic alopecia is found to occur mainly in Western civilization or those who have adopted the ways of Western civilization, meaning that there may be dietary practices that contribute to hair loss and therefore giving hope to the possibility that diet could control not only temporary hair loss, but androgenetic alopecia as well.

Doctors and scientists are studying DHT production in the body to understand it more thoroughly. There is an obvious link to hair loss and prostatic health and this only increases the pace of hair loss discoveries. Most treatments for prostatic diseases such as benign prostatic hyperplasia (BPH) also have the pleasant side affect of growing hair on the heads of those taking it. With the pace of research and discoveries today, there is a great deal of optimism in the field of hair loss prevention. Hair is an important part of our dress and appearance, therefore a large part of our self-esteem. It is likely that there are answers for your situation presently or coming in the near future.

Remember, the restoration of hair growth is not an overnight process. The process takes time regardless of the method chosen. Be patient and follow as much of the advice given by professionals as possible. Keep in mind that the body is a system, and it is the abuse of this system by food intake and environmental causes that lead to most common hair loss. Through returning the body back to its natural state, hair growth can be restored. Good health to you *Restore your Beautiful Hair!*

RESOURCES FOR HAIR CARE AND HAIR LOSS PREVENTION

Hair Loss Control Center
http://www.hlcc.com

Hair Club for women and men
http://www.hairclub.com

Bosley
http://bosley.com

Trichotillomania
http://trich.org

Products for hair Loss Prevention

Amway
http://tiny.cc/mkq1bw

Hair Loss Control Center
http://hlcconline.com

Tropical Traditions Coconut oil and other products
http://tinyurl.com/82o62hp

Where to find Great Hair

Extensions Plus
http://extensions-plus.com

Dry Me Quick Dryer Cap

This cap will help dry your Quick! 50-80% ***QUICKER!***

Save time and money and go green reduce energy cost!
http://drymequickdryercap.com

AUTHOR

George Greene knows and loves beautiful and healthy hair. Enjoying over twenty-five years as licensed Master Cosmetologist, Salon Owner, Cosmetology Educator, Hair Stylist and entrepreneur has allowed him to witness the devastating affect of women hair loss. "Restore My Beautiful Hair" gives you proven and practical solutions to help women hair loss suffers restore their hair. If you are suffering hair loss, hair thinning, or you want to prevent having to suffer this shameful experience, this book is for you. You can *RESTORE YOUR BEAUTIFUL HAIR"!*

Contact Information:

http://restoremybeautifulhair.com
http://facebook.com/GeorgeGreenwayzz
http://twitter.com/GeorgeGreene
http://drymequickdryercap.com
http://george-green.com

George Greene ****678-818-4333

Restore My Beautiful Hair

Author George Greene

Are you one of 60 million women of color suffering hair thinning or hair loss? Are you tired of embarrassing hair moments? Are you disappointed with your hair? Are you sick and tired of losing your hair?

You are now holding in your hands," Restore My Beautiful Hair", practical, proven and preventable SOLUTIONS you can use NOW to restore your beautiful hair. Yes there is hope and you can start today restoring, repairing and re-growing your beautiful hair. This informative and practical guide was written by a Master Cosmetologist, Hair Loss Specialist and Educator with over twenty-five years in the beauty industry. Mr. Greene has worked with one of the world's leading hair restoration companies and can share with you how to overcome your hair challenges."Restore My Beautiful Hair" will give you a better understanding why women of color victims of and contributors to their hair loss, possibly without their knowledge.

What causes hair loss and hair thinning? Can my hair loss or thinning be prevented? Are there solutions I can start now that will stop and prevent hair loss? What products are best to use for my hair type and texture? How can I grow my natural hair?

Your hope to restore your hair lies here on these pages and this information is for you and all women and little women of color. If you want to restore your hair to it's healthy radiance and stop losing your, start here! Take this guide home with you and share this information.

Learn about topical treatments, scalp exfoliants, DHT Inhibitors, nutritional supplements for your hair, Trichotillomania, medications, low light laser therapy, surgical and non-surgical solutions for your hair. Do not be mis- lead, mis- informed or confused you now have the answers you need to, "Restore My Beautiful Hair".

RESTORE MY BEAUTIFUL HAIR author George Greene

www.ingramcontent.com/pod-product-compliance
Lightning Source LLC
Chambersburg PA
CBHW050343290526
45785CB00006B/2617